VEGETARIANISM

A Beguinner's Guide

by

PAUL POWELL

TABLE OF CONTENTS

Introduction 4

Chapter 1: What Is Vegetarianism? 6

Chapter 2: How To Transition To A Vegetarian Diet.......... 13

Chapter 3: Supplementation Guidelines........................... 20

Chapter 4: Recipes... 23

Conclusion 27

INTRODUCTION

Today, more and more people are suffering from what is called affluence diseases or sicknesses caused by ever increasing wealth. How's wealth bad for people? For one, wealth comes at a price, which is usually ever-increasing workloads and ever decreasing time for anything else. As such, more and more people are finding it hard to find a chance to take care of themselves via exercise and preparing healthy food for daily consumption. And because their free time continues to erode, fast foods continue to become more of the norm in most countries, especially the most industrialised ones.

Vegetarianism is a way of life that is beneficial for everyone concerned: you, the people around you, and the animals around you. In what ways? That's what you'll find out in this book. And more than the benefits, you'll learn how to successfully transition from your predominantly carnivore lifestyle to a vegetarian one together with a couple of deliciously healthy recipes to start you off on your journey towards great health.

If you're ready, turn the page and let's begin!

CHAPTER 1:

WHAT IS VEGETARIANISM?

"I'm not a vegetarian because I love animals. I'm a vegetarian because I hate plants."

–A. Whitney Brown

For many people, there is a lot of confusion regarding the word "vegetarian". Vegetarian refers to a lifestyle or a diet that is plant-based and avoids the consumption of meat or anything made or derived from animals such as dairy products and oil.

As food, vegetarianism can be classified into four types namely Ovo-vegetarian, lacto Vegetarian, Lacto-Ovo vegetarian, and vegan. An Ovo vegetarian diet is one wherein consumption of eggs (Ovo) is allowed. As you may have already guessed, a Lacto-vegetarian diet allows the consumption of milk or dairy products like yoghurt, cheese, and milk. Obviously, a lacto-ovo-vegetarian is one where consumption of both eggs and dairy products are allowed. And lastly, there's the vegan diet. This diet is the most hardcore of all the types of vegetarian diets because here, no animal-based or animal derived products are consumed.

While being a vegetarian is mostly about what is eating, it can also extend the people's Lifestyles as a whole. In particular, veganism is a lifestyle that avoids consuming or using any products that exploit or harm animals in the process such as leather jackets, fur coats, and cosmetic products that were first tested on animals, among others.

So why would people go to Such Great Lengths to avoid consuming meat and other animal-derived stuff? Considering that it's very hard and cumbersome to avoid eating meat and many other food items made from animals, living a vegetarian lifestyle mainly eating a vegetarian diet can be very hard and practical for most people.

Brief History

As a practice, vegetarianism started as far back as during the ancient Indian and Greek civilisations. In most civilisations, the diet was tied to the principle of nonviolence when it comes to relating to animals, which is referred to as Ahimsa in Indian culture. This was promulgated by their philosophers and major religious groups.

Vegetarian almost became extinct in Europe once the Roman Empire became Christian between the 4th and 6th centuries. The only way it survived as a practice in Europe is when different orders of monks during the Medieval ages prohibited the eating or consumption of meat due to religious or ascetic reasons. Many of these monks, however, we're not total vegetarians but rather more like pescatarians, which substituted fish for meat in their diets. During the Renaissance period in Europe, vegetarianism came back with a vengeance and became very popular as a practice from the 19th to the 20th centuries.

Reasons For Going Vegetarian

There are lots of scientific evidence that makes an adamant case for eating a vegetarian diet. In particular, adopting a vegetarian diet can significantly improve our health. When you look at it, the federal government of the United States even suggests that the ideal diet is one where most of the calories consumed for the day are derived from plant-based sources. Ever wondered why?

This is because of the many scientific evidence that points to meat consumption, or at least excessive amounts of it, as the single biggest reason for many serious health conditions today including heart disease. Going vegetarian can help to radically bring down our risks for many serious health conditions such as high blood pressure, obesity, coronary artery disease, and certain types of cancers.

Healthy Weight

When you take a look at the diet of most people in the world today, it is quite concerning. Why? It's because the typical diet most people follow is one that is very high in bad fats, also known as saturated fats, as well as highly processed food. Worse, search diets are very low in complex carbohydrates and plant-based food items. Hence, many people in the world today are obese, and the number just keeps increasing.

Adopting a vegetarian diet helps people achieve a healthy weight because apart from it being low in fat, which contains more than twice the calories for the same amount of carbohydrates or proteins, a vegetarian diet is one that is also rich in dietary fibre. One study conducted between 1986 to 1992 found on average, the study's participants lost around 24 pounds within 12 months and even better, we're able to maintain the healthy weight that they were able to achieve even five years after the study. The best thing about it? The studies subjects didn't have to monitor their caloric consumption strictly. They just ate naturally and abundantly.

Daily Energy And Mental Performance

A vegetarian diet is one that's very high in complex carbohydrates and dietary fibre, both of which help increase energy levels and improve mental performance by reducing brain fog and mental sluggishness. So if you want to be able to do more during the day, consider going vegetarian.

Long Life

Do you find your life to be a very satisfying and beautiful one and do you want to live such a life for a long time? If that's the case, then you will surely want to go vegetarian. Do you want proof? Consider the Japanese and particularly, those that live in Okinawa. Any study that was featured in the book the Real Age Diet written by Michael Roizen, it was shown that this particular group of people enjoyed the highest life expectancy in their country and one of the largest all over the world. The study also noted that the reason for this is their diet which is composed primarily of a plant-based product such as soy, fruits, vegetables high in dietary fibre, and complex carbohydrates.

For Women

A vegetarian diet is one that is rich in phytoestrogens. These are compounds that tend to copy the actions of the women's hormone oestrogen as well as help in balancing women's progesterone and oestrogen levels. These two help to reduce incidences of problematic transitions towards menopause. In particular, soy is the best plant-based food regarding phytoestrogen content, so a plant-based diet that's high in soy helps in reducing problems that come as women transition towards menopause later in life.

Ethics

For many vegetarians, their reasons for living the lifestyle is more than just their personal benefits – it's also about animals' lives. For them, eating a meat-based diet is one that supports being cruel to animals. If you've seen an animal being slaughtered for food, you'll get where vegetarians are coming from on this one.

Another ethical reason for going vegetarian is to help more people have something to eat. How's that? Raising more and more livestock require more crops for their consumption. And most of the time, this keeps many poor and hungry people from getting enough food for themselves. By going vegetarian, the demand for livestock may go down and along with it, the animals' demand for crops. That can set more plants free for poor and hungry people to eat.

And lastly, eating meat contributes to the continuous erosion of our planet. Why? It's because the commercial raising of livestock takes a lot of resources such as land, energy and water, to name a few. As more and more animal needs to be raised, more energy, land and water are consumed, which contribute to the faster degeneration of our planet. So when people go vegetarian, demand for livestock decreases and we slow down our world's decay.

CHAPTER 2:

HOW TO TRANSITION TO A VEGETARIAN DIET

Make no mistake about it, going vegetarian isn't kidded stuff. It will challenge your fortitude, self-control, and willpower. Especially if you love eating meat, it may be very challenging at the beginning requiring every ounce of strength you have just to transition. But the good news is it is possible in overtime; the development becomes easier and easier until the vegetarian diet is already second nature to you.

It has been said that the shortest distance between two points is a straight line. That is true. And in the case of going from a meat-based diet to a vegetarian one, it looks to be as simple as ditching meat in favour of plant-based food. Often, however, the easiest and shortest route is the hardest where many men and women when to give up in the middle of the journey. As such, the best way to transition from a meat-based diet to a vegetarian one is to take a seemingly longer route with several stops in between. It may take longer, but it will not be as overwhelming as taking the shortest route to becoming a vegetarian. As such, your risks for quitting and dropping out will be significantly less and your chances of successfully transitioning a vegetarian diet become significantly higher. Let's take a look at the different ways you can start transitioning from your current carnivorous diet to a vegetarian one.

Assess Your Current Diet

As with any journey, you need first to know where you currently are to plot out a route that will take you to your destination. In this case, it's going vegetarian.

Well, it's obvious that you are currently eating a diet that's not vegetarian, it is important to assess how much of a carnivore you are before setting off for your vegetarian journey. Are you on a ketogenic diet, where most if not all of your calories come from meat, dairy, and fat? Or are you already eating some fruits, vegetables, grains, or rice in your diet together with meat and fish? If you're eating mostly meat and meat-derived foods, expect that your journey towards becoming a full-fledged vegetarian will take longer compared to if you're already eating some more moderate amounts of plant-based food.

Set Realistic Goals

Nothing else can be as devastating for your vegetarian transition efforts than setting goals that are too lofty or unrealistic. You know about the same the higher you fly, the harder you fall? If you set your goals too high, you will not reach them, but because of the massive efforts you've already put in, your disappointment or discouragement can be just as extensive or intense. As such, the chances are high that you will abandon your goals altogether.

So when it comes to transitioning to become a full-fledged veteran, don't just set one big massive goal such as becoming a total vegetarian. Set smaller and more realistic and achievable goals that can serve as stepping stones by which you can achieve your primary goal of becoming a full vegetarian. How does this look like?

Examples of setting smaller realistic goals that help you eventually transition into becoming a total vegetarian include not eating pork for the first month then avoiding beef together with pork on the second month, then adding chicken to the list of forbidden foods on the 3rd month and so on until you have successfully transitioned to a vegetarian diet.

Baby Steps

After setting smaller and more realistic goals, it's time to break them down even further into actionable steps that you can take to achieve these aims. Why do you need to do this?

Remember what I wrote earlier about going for one big but the unrealistic goal? In particular, how it can become a guarantee for failure by giving you a massive sense of disappointment or discouragement that will make you quit in the middle of the journey. Taking baby steps is the exact opposite.

By breaking down your realistic goals into several smaller and actionable steps, you give yourself the opportunity to accomplish many small victories. And as your small victories continue to pile up, you can become more and more encouraged and pumped up to take on more or bigger actions that can yield even more major successes and victories. Think of your morale as a snowball that starts out small as it begins to roll down a hill and becomes huge by the time it gets to the bottom because along the way; it was able to accumulate more and more snow. By experiencing more and smaller victories, you enable yourself to take on much bigger risks and achieve even more major victories until you are finally able to transition towards full vegetarianism.

How do these baby steps look like regarding transitioning towards vegetarianism? Let's consider the smaller, more realistic goals we used earlier as an example:

Goal #1: Stop eating pork for the first 30 days.
• Week 1: Talk to your family and friends about your desire to go vegetarian and to ask their help and support;
• Week 2: Stop buying pork chops during your weekly groceries;
• Week 3: Stop eating at your favourite restaurant, Peter Porker's Pork Haven; and
• Week 4: Before taking a seat in any restaurant, check the menu first if other tasty dishes don't involve pork.

Goal #2: Stop eating pork and beef in the second month.
• Week 1: Stop buying beef jerky;
• Week 2: Stop buying meat for lunch/dinner;
• Week 3: Watch a video of cows being slaughtered to feel a strong sense of disdain for eating meat; and
• Week 4: Start eating a cup of any vegetable during breakfast.

Are you getting it now? I won't give you an exact plan for you to follow regarding actionable steps and realistic goals because each and every one of us has different situations, characteristics, personalities. Only you and the people closest to you know you best and that such, you'll be in the best position to set you're smaller realistic goals and baby steps two words transitioning entirely to vegetarianism.

Plan Well

There is a wise saying about how failing to plan is the same as planning to fail. When it comes to transitioning successfully to a vegetarian diet or lifestyle, you will need to think ahead, anticipate possible challenges or obstacles, and come up with plans on how to overcome those expected challenges or obstacles. If regret comes only in the end, then assuming only arrives in the beginning.

One of the best ways to start planning for your transition is journaling. Start by keeping a journal of all the foods that you eat every day and how you felt before eating them. Yes, it can be very cumbersome at first but believe me, it will give you powerful insights as to why you eat what you are eating now. There was even a study that showed journaling as a very powerful change in diet that led to other significant variations in another feeding, all of which eventually resulted in healthy and lasting weight loss for all of that study's participants.

When you start journaling about the foods that you eat every day, the very first thing that changes about you is awareness. You start to become more and more mindful of the things that you eat and often, mindless eating is the culprit when it comes to poor eating habits and choices. Often too, simply being aware of what is consumed is enough to empower people to choose healthy food instead of unhealthy ones.

CHAPTER 3:

SUPPLEMENTATION GUIDELINES

W hy did indeed true that a vegetarian diet is one that can do much for your General Health, personal and looks, it's not perfect. I mean, nothing is. Like a diet or a general eating plan, the vegetarian diet also tends to be deficient in some vital minerals and vitamins even if you eat truckloads of only fruits and vegetables. But the good news is, these potential deficiencies should not be a hindrance to your transition into vegetarianism and experience its many incredible benefits. You can supplement your diet to avoid mineral and vitamin deficiencies.

Calcium

This is one of the minerals vegetarians tend to be deficient in. More than just helping make your teeth and bones stronger, calcium also helps regarding blood clotting and Contracting your muscles. Chronic deficiency of calcium may lead to weak bones, also known as osteoporosis, which increases the risks for fractures and tooth decay.

How much calcium should you be getting every day? Ideally, you should be going with this least 1000 up to 1300 mg as an adult. As a vegetarian, especially if you're not a Lacto-vegetarian, you'll be skipping out on the best source of the mineral, which is milk. And to get the same amount of calcium from plants, you would need to eat a lot.

Iron

Another essential mineral that is deficient in most vegetarians is iron. Primarily because this mineral is very much abundant in the very thing that vegetarians abhor kama which me and in particular, beef. Iron is responsible for the efficient delivery of oxygen to the body's cells.

Chronic deficiency in this mineral increases your risk for suffering from anaemia. The symptoms of anaemia include getting easily fatigued, frequently feeling fatigued, peptic ulcers, and a general feeling of weakness. And as I mentioned earlier, the bad news is that you can only get enough iron from meat. Fortunately, you can make up for such deficiency by eating iron-rich plants taking iron supplements. Ideally, should be getting 8.7 mg or 14.8 mg if you're a man or a woman, respectively.

Vitamin B12

This particular vitamin is essential to maintain proper metabolism optimal nervous system and brain health, healthy blood formation, and proper metabolism. Even if you're not a vegetarian, you can still suffer deficiencies of this vitamin because they can only be found in archaea and bacteria. As such, the only real option for you to get enough of this essential vitamin is through supplementation.

CHAPTER 4:

RECIPES

Most people who fail to stick to their diets did not do so because of bland or unhealthy tasting food. I mean it's bad enough to ditch the meat and anything related to it but it's a different thing altogether to substitute them with crappy food. I, therefore, conclude that one of the biggest secrets to successfully transitioning to and staying in a vegetarian diet is delicious vegetarian recipes.

And that is what this last chapter is all about. I will give you several delicious vegetarian recipes that will not just help you become vegetarian but will make you love it.

Sunrise Tofu Breakfast Delight

Ingredients:

• A large clove of minced garlic;

• A package tofu drained of water;

• A small diced onion;

• Chopped small tomatoes, two pieces;

• Half a teaspoon of cumin;

• Pepper to taste;

• Turmeric, ¼ teaspoon;

• Water, two tablespoons; and

• Wheat free soy sauce, 1 to 2 tablespoons.

Instructions:

• In a saucepan, heat your soy sauce and water before mixing in the garlic and stirring. Threw in the turmeric, cumin and onions and sautéed until your onions turn tender.

• Mix in the tofu. Let the mixture simmer for up to 6 minutes before tossing the chopped tomatoes in. Continue cooking for one more minute.

• Remove the mixture from heat and for a fuller breakfast, eat it warm together with brown rice.

Beanie Burger Lunch Treat

Ingredients:

• A small jalapeno pepper, minced;

• A small onion;

• A tablespoon of olive oil;

• Chilli powder, two teaspoons;

• Cooked and mashed black beans, 2 cups;

• Cuming ¼ teaspoon;

• Half a cup of bread crumbs;

• Half a cup of corn niblets;

• Half a cup of whole wheat flour;

• Half a medium red pepper diced;

• Half a teaspoon of dried oregano;

• Half a teaspoon of salt;

• Minced fresh parsley, two tablespoons; and

• Minced garlic, two cloves.

Instructions:

• Over the medium-high heat, sauté together in oil the oregano, onion, garlic and jalapeno pepper until your onions turn translucent.

• Add the red peppers in and sauté for another 2 minutes or until the peppers turn tender. When done, take away from heat and set the mixture aside.

• After mashing your black beans, mix it with the cumin, vegetables, salt, breadcrumbs, chilli powder, and parsley. From this combination, shape out five burger patties of equal sizes, which you'll coat with flour on all sides.

• Fry your beanie burger patties on a pan that're slightly oiled for 5 to 10 minutes on medium-high heat until both sides are cooked well.

Delicious Diet Spinach Salad Dinner

Ingredients:

• A medium carrot, shredded;

• A tablespoon of balsamic vinegar;

• Chopped spinach, 2 cups;

• Half a bell pepper;

• Half a cup of Broccoli, cooked and cooled;

• Half a cup of chopped tomato;

• Half a cup of shredded cabbage; and

• Salt and pepper to taste.

Instructions:

• This salad is very complicated to prepare. Toss and combine everything well. That's it. Very confusing, eh?

CONCLUSION

Now that you know what vegetarianism is, the many incredible benefits it holds for you in waiting, how to transition to vegetarianism successfully, how to make sure you get enough important vitamins and minerals as a vegetarian, and a couple of deliciously healthy recipes for the whole day, what should you do next?

It's simple. Knowing is only half the battle. The other half is action or the application of knowledge. The next step, therefore, is to take action and apply the things you've learned here by planning out your route towards vegetarianism, learning more deliciously healthy vegetarian recipes, and start reducing your meat consumption today and gradually reduce it even more. Remember, it doesn't have to be fast. Take baby steps, so you start experiencing many small victories and eventually be able to transition into vegetarianism successfully.

Here's to your health and success, my friend! Cheers!